SMOO

JARED

Smoothies for Athletes and Weight Loss

Keep Healthy With Green Smoothies for Weight Loss

By: Jared Boulder

9781632874702

PUBLISHERS NOTES

Disclaimer – Speedy Publishing, LLC

This publication is intended to provide helpful and informative material. It is not intended to diagnose, treat, cure, or prevent any health problem or condition, nor is intended to replace the advice of a physician. No action should be taken solely on the contents of this book. Always consult your physician or qualified health-care professional on any matters regarding your health and before adopting any suggestions in this book or drawing inferences from it.

The author and publisher specifically disclaim all responsibility for any liability, loss or risk, personal or otherwise, which is incurred as a consequence, directly or indirectly, from the use or application of any contents of this book.

Any and all product names referenced within this book are the trademarks of their respective owners. None of these owners have sponsored, authorized, endorsed, or approved this book.

Always read all information provided by the manufacturers' product labels before using their products. The author and publisher are not responsible for claims made by manufacturers.

This book was originally printed before 2014. This is an adapted reprint by Speedy Publishing, LLC with newly updated content designed to help readers with much more accurate and timely information and data.

Speedy Publishing, LLC

40 E Main Street,

Newark

Delaware

19711

Contact Us: 1-888-248-4521

Website: http://www.speedypublishing.com

REPRINTED Paperback Edition: ISBN: 9781632874702

Manufactured in the United States of America

DEDICATION

This book is dedicated to my family and my dear friend Rasheed. Without their support I would never have had the courage to start writing.

TABLE OF CONTENTS

CHAPTER 1- INTRODUCTION TO SMOOTHIES & FRUIT JUICES

A FUN and EASY way to get more vitamins & minerals into your diet is by drinking freshly made fruit juices, vegetable juices, and by blending thick and frothy smoothies and shakes from frozen fruit.

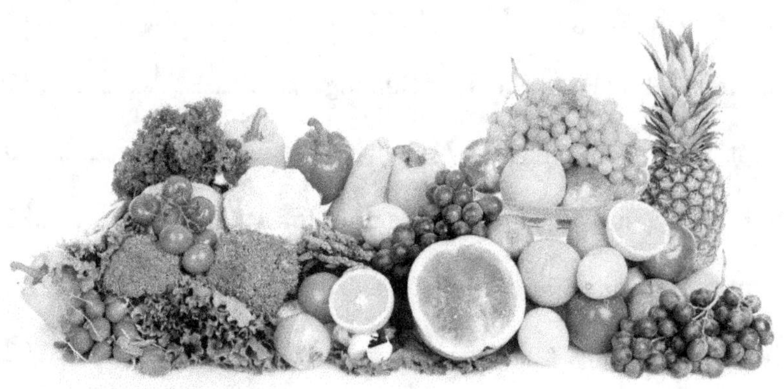

A friend of mine describes drinking freshly made fruit juices like this:

"If you have never taken a mouthful of cantaloupe juice or strawberry juice mixed with apple, you simply have not lived. Blueberry juice is a taste of liquid heaven."

Freshly made juices are a tremendous source of bio-available vitamins and minerals which are the partners of enzymes and co-enzymes. Vitamins activate enzymes and without vitamins, enzymes could not carry out their work, and we could not live.

Enzymes act as catalysts in hundreds of thousands of chemical reactions that take place throughout your body, and are essential for digesting, absorbing and converting food into body tissue. Enzymes produce energy at the cellular level and are critical for most of the metabolic activities taking place in your body every second of every day.

Another benefit of drinking fresh juices and smoothies is that your body can absorb MORE of the vitamins and minerals than if you were to eat the fruits and vegetables whole! Many of the nutrients are TRAPPED in the fiber and by blending fruits and vegetables, you break down the fiber and release the vital nutrients.

Example:

When you eat a raw carrot, you are only able to assimilate a small percentage of the available beta carotene. When a carrot is juiced, removing the fiber, a LARGE percentage of the beta carotene can be assimilated by your body.

Of course, you still need to eat whole produce because fiber is also an important part of your daily diet.

Meeting you or your children's need for energy and nutrients is essential for good health. Children who do not meet their needs for energy may stop growing and gaining weight. In severe situations, they can develop a condition which is life threatening called protein energy malnutrition. Vitamins and minerals are only required in very small amounts, but a diet insufficient in these can cause SEVERE deficiency diseases.

You may be showing signs of malnutrition if you ...

*   feel tired and weak.

* • feel like you never have the energy to clean your home, make meals or even do the dishes.
* have difficulty losing or gaining weight.
* can't easily get to sleep.
* feel stressed and/or nervous.
* feel drowsy during the day.
* sometimes can't concentrate, you're mind feels numb, or you get confused easily.
* have problems with your digestion.
* have constipation and/or hard dry stools.
* have mood swings, or get easily upset.
* don't have patience for anything.
* sometimes feel depressed.
* have overly dry or oily skin.
* sometimes have nausea and/or abdominal pain.
* have annoying eye twitches.
* bruise easily.
* have muscle cramps and/or low back pain.
* sometimes get cracks and sores in the corners of your mouth.
* notice that your nails have become thin and/or brittle.
* are losing your hair.
* have water retention.
* have uncontrollable temper outbursts.
* don't eat a well-balanced nutritious diet EVERY DAY

Natural vitamins are found only in living things, that is, plants and animals. Your body, with a few exceptions, can't manufacture vitamins. They must be supplied in your food or in dietary supplements but supplements can't replace food, especially fruits and vegetables which provide thousands of substances, some of which have well-known functions, and some whose roles in the human body are not yet understood or recognized.

Vitamins and Minerals ... ...

* reduce your risk of getting a stroke or heart attack
* strengthen your nails
* improve your hair condition, strength and growth by providing certain essential nutrients to the hair follicle
* beautify your skin by keeping it smooth, soft and disease-free
* provide essential compounds that are necessary for growth, health, normal metabolism and physical well-being! Without them, you would die
* promote normal growth and development
* maintain bone density and strength
* regulate blood clotting
* help in the function of nerves and muscles, including regulating a normal heart beat

When it comes to choosing a healthy diet for their children, many parents don't realize the important role that beverages play. For example, fruit flavored drinks and soft drinks are not a substitute for real fruit. Many of these drinks only contain 10% real fruit juice. The very best drinks are made from whole fruit and you can make great fruity healthy drinks at home.

How to Make Homemade Fruit and Vegetable Juices

1. You'll need an inexpensive juice machine.
2. All fruits and vegetables should be juiced raw.
3. Small seeded fruit, such as watermelon and pears, may be juiced with their seeds with the exception of papaya and apple seeds. Orange and grapefruit seeds might impart a

bitter taste to your juice. Remove the large pits from fruits like peaches and nectarines, etc.

4. Peel all fruits and vegetables that are not organically grown because the peel is where most of the chemical residues can be found. While most skins of organically grown fruits and vegetables may be left on, with the exception of waxed produce, the skins of pineapples, kiwis, oranges, grapefruits and papaya should be removed.

5. Choose fresh ripe produce. Rubbery vegetables, bruised fruit, wilted greens and over or under-ripe fruits will produce juices that are neither tasty nor healthful.

6. Cut the fruits or vegetables into pieces that will fit into the mouth of your juice machine. Turn the juice machine on and push the pieces through the mouth of the juicer. As you juice, pulp will collect in a large receptacle. If you don't clean the pulp out right away, it will develop a

7. sour odor and tiny gnats and fruit flies may appear after 8 to 10 hours.

8. It is best to drink freshly made juices within one day.

5 Steps to Making the Perfect Smoothie

1. Put the fruit in the blender first. Make sure that the items are smaller than a golf ball so they will blend completely. Add the liquid ingredients next.

2. Fasten the lid and press the start button. Use high speed for about 20- 30 seconds.

3. Stop the blender and check to see if the ingredients are well blended. Sometimes the frozen fruit will jam under the blade. If there is jammed fruit, use a spatula to unjam the fruit, and blend again.

4. Once the mixture is evenly blended, slowly add two ice cubes through the opening of the blender lid. Keep adding one or two ice cubes at a time until the blender sounds

smooth instead of gravelly. If your blender is not strong enough to blend ice cubes, omit the ice and substitute just enough ice cold water so that the shake will have a milkshake consistency.

5. If the shake/smoothie is too thin, add more fruit or ice. If it's too thick, add more liquid.

Smoothie and Shake Tips

A smoothie is basically a blended fruit drink. The best-tasting smoothies are made from fruit that is fresh or frozen, and not canned.

All smoothies begin with a liquid base. This can be orange juice, milk or another liquid.

You can make a frostier drink by freezing fresh fruit before making a smoothie.

Smoothies are best when they're fresh out of the blender, but they can be frozen the night before, as well – just remove the smoothie from the freezer about an hour before drinking.

You can replace a meal with a smoothie or shake by adding a scoop of high-quality protein powder and a tbsp. of high-quality olive or flax oil.

CHAPTER 2- HOMEMADE BEAUTY RECIPES

Avocado Facial

Avocado is a naturally rich moisturizer. Mash the meat of the avocado into a creamy texture. Massage into the face and neck. Leave on for 15 minutes and gently rinse off.

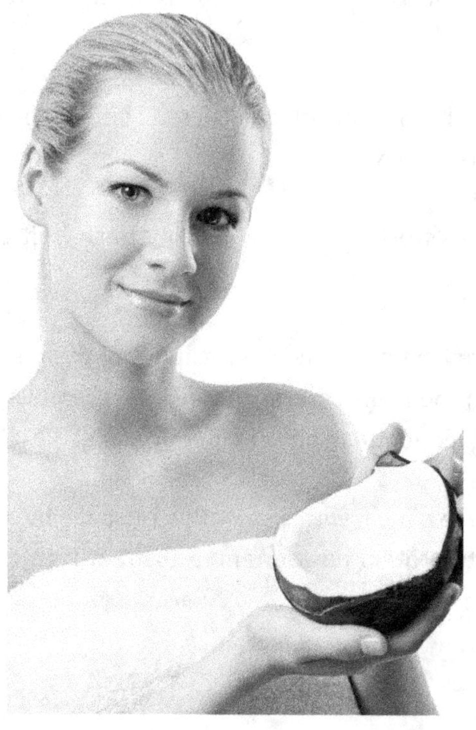

Facial Mask

Squeeze half a lemon and mix the juice with one beaten egg white. Leave on your face overnight or, for a quick pick-me-up, just 15 minutes. Splash warm water on your face to rinse. It helps to removes blotches, because the lemon works as a bleaching agent.

Egg & Honey Mask

Mix together 1 tablespoon honey, 1 egg yolk, 1/2 teaspoon almond oil and 1 tablespoon yogurt. Honey stimulates and smoothes, egg and almond oil penetrate and moisturize, and yogurt refines and tightens pores.

Cornmeal Facial Mask

Two tablespoons of cornmeal mixed with enough water to make a thick paste makes a great inexpensive facial mask. Gently apply to face and wash off.

Lighten Circles under Eyes

To lighten dark circles under your eyes, wrap a grated raw potato in cheesecloth and apply to eyelids for 15-20 minutes. Wipe off residue and apply an eye cream.

Egg, Avocado & Mud Facial Mask

(best for oilier skin types)

Clay is available in powder form at any health food store. Mix 1 tbsp. dry clay with 1 egg yolk, 1/4 of a mashed avocado and enough witch hazel to create a smooth mixture. Mud dries excess sebum while the egg yolk and avocado replenish lost moisture. Witch hazel tones.

Egg & Olive Oil Hair Mask

Mix two whole eggs with four tablespoons of olive oil. Smooth through hair. Wrap head with plastic wrap, and leave in hair for 10 minutes. Rinse well.

Fruit Smoothie Hair Mask

Blend 1/2 a banana, 1/4 avocado, 1/4 cantaloupe, 1 tablespoon wheat germ oil and 1 tablespoon yogurt. For extra conditioning, squeeze in the contents of a vitamin E capsule. Leave in hair for 15 minutes.

Facial Exfoliater

2 heaped tsp. fine oatmeal 1 tsp. baking soda

Combine ingredients, and add enough water to make a paste. Apply to skin and rub gently. Rinse and gently pat dry.

Banana Wrinkle Fighter

Banana is wonderful as an anti-wrinkle treatment. Mash 1/4 banana until very creamy. Spread all over face and leave for 15-20 minutes before rinsing off with warm water followed by a dash of cold. Gently pat dry.

Grape Cleanser

Grape juice makes an excellent cleanser for any skin type. Simply split one or two large grapes, remove pips and rub the flesh over face and neck.

Rinse off with cool water.

CHAPTER 3- FASTING FOR WEIGHT LOSS

Loss of weight indicates, almost guarantees, that detoxification and healing is occurring. I can't stress this too much. Of all the things I find my patients seem to misunderstand or forget after being told, it is that they can't heal in a rapid manner without getting smaller. This reality is especially hard for the family and friends of someone who is fasting, who will say, "you're looking terrible dear, so thin. Your skin is hanging on your bones.

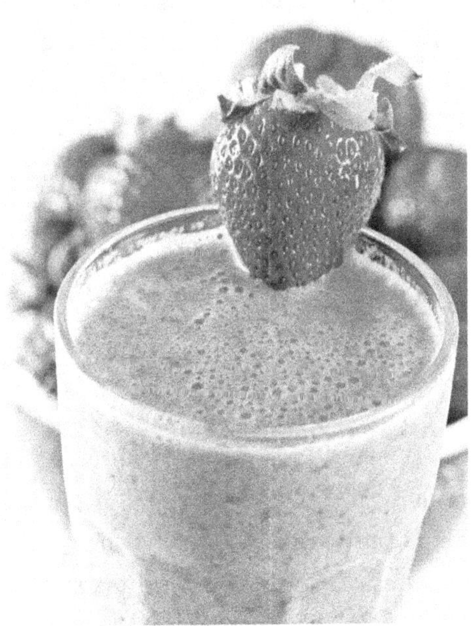

You're not eating enough protein or nutrient food to be healthy and you must eat more or you're going to develop serious deficiencies. You don't have any energy, you must be getting sicker. You're doing the wrong thing, obviously. You have less energy and look worse every day. Go and see a doctor before it is too late." To succeed with friends like this, a faster has to be a mighty self-determined person with a powerful ability to disagree with others.

Medical personnel claim that rapid weight loss often causes dangerous deficiencies; these deficiencies force the person to overeat and regain even more weight afterward. This is largely untrue, though there is one true aspect to it: a fasted, detoxified body becomes a much more efficient digester and assimilator, extracting a lot more nutrition from the same amount food is used to eat. If, after extended fasting a person returns to eating the same number of calories as they did before; they will gain weight even more rapidly than before they stated fasting.

When fasting for weight loss, the only way to keep the weight off is to greatly reform the diet; to go on, and stay on, a diet made up largely of non- starchy, watery fruits and vegetables, limited quantities of cooked food, and very limited amounts of highly concentrated food sources like cereals and cooked legumes. Unless, of course, after fasting, one's lifestyle involves much very hard physical labor or exercise. I've had a few obese fasters become quite angry with me for this reason; they hoped to get thin through fasting and after the fast, to resume overeating with complete irresponsibility as before, without weight gain.

People also fear weight loss during fasting because they fear becoming anorexic or bulimic. They won't! A person who abstains from eating for the purpose of improving their health, in order to prevent or treat illness, or even one who fasts for weight loss will not develop an eating disorder. Eating disorders mean eating compulsively because of a distorted body image. Anorexics and bulimics have obsessions with the thinner-is-better school of thought.

The anorexic looks at their emaciated frame in the mirror and thinks they are fat! This is the distorted perception of a very insecure person badly in need of therapy. A bulimic, on the other hand stuffs themselves, usually with bad food, and then purges it by vomiting, or with laxatives. Anorexics and bulimics are not accelerating the healing potential of their bodies; these are life threatening conditions. Fasters are genuinely trying to enhance their survival potential.

Occasionally a neurotic individual with a pre-existing eating disorder will become obsessed with fasting and colon cleansing as a justification to legitimize their compulsion. During my career while monitoring hundreds of fasters, I've known two of these. I discourage them from fasting or colon cleansing, and refuse to assist them, because they carry the practices to absurd extremes, and contribute to bad press about natural medicine by ending up in the emergency ward of a hospital with an intravenous feeding tube in their arm.

CHAPTER 4- RAW FOOD DIETS FOR HEALING

Next in declining order of healing effectiveness is what I call a raw food healing diet or cleansing diet. It consists of those very same watery fruits and non-starchy vegetables one juices or makes into vegetable broths, but eaten whole and raw. Heating food does two harmful things: it destroys many vitamins, enzymes and other nutritional elements and it makes many foods much harder to digest.

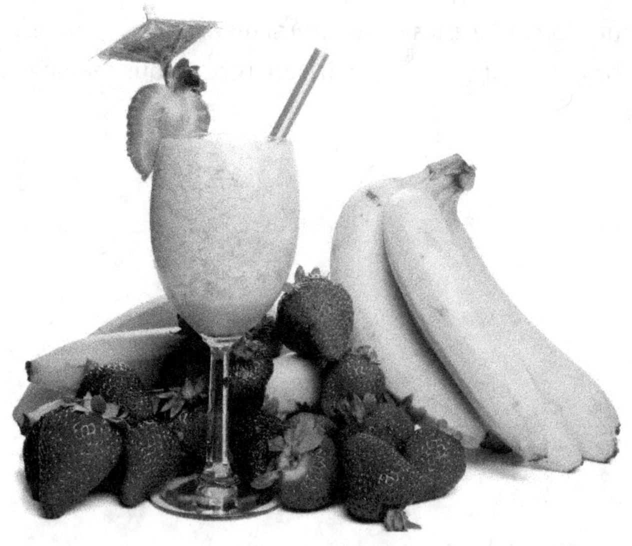

So no cooked vegetables or fruits are allowed because to maintain health on this limited regimen it is essential that every possible vitamin and enzyme present in the food be available for digestion. Even though still raw, no starchy or fatty vegetables or fruits are allowed that contain concentrated calories like potatoes, winter squash, avocados, sweet potatoes, fresh raw corn, dates, figs, raisins, or bananas. And naturally, no salad dressings containing vegetable oils or (raw) ground seeds are allowed nor are raw grains or other raw concentrated energy sources.

When a person starts this diet they will at first experience considerable weight loss because it is difficult to extract a large number of calories from these foods (though I have seen people actually gain weight on a pure melon diet, so much sugar do these fruits have, and well-chewed watermelon seeds are very nourishing). Eating even large quantities of only raw fruit and raw non-starchy vegetables results in a slow but steady healing process about 10 to 20 percent as rapid as water fasting.

A raw food cleansing diet has several huge advantages. It is possible to maintain this regimen and regularly do non-strenuous work for many months, even a year or more without experiencing massive weight loss and, more important to some people, without suffering the extremes of low blood sugar, weakness and loss of ability to concentrate that happen when water fasting. Someone on a raw food cleanse will have periods of lowered energy and strong cravings for more concentrated foods, but if they have the self-discipline to not break their cleansing process they can accomplish a great deal of healing while still maintaining more or less normal (though slower paced) life activities. However, almost no one on this diet is able to sustain an extremely active life-style involving hard physical labor or competitive sports.

And from the very beginning someone on a raw food cleanse must be willing and able to lie down and rest any time they feel tired or unable to face their responsibilities. Otherwise they will inevitably succumb to the mental certainty that their feelings of exhaustion or overwhelm can be immediately solved by eating some concentrated food to "give them energy." Such low-energy states will, however, pass quickly after a brief nap or rest.

Something else gradually happens to a body when on such a diet. Do you recall that I mentioned that after my own long fast I began to get more "mileage" out of my food. A cleansed, healed body becomes far more efficient at digestion and assimilation; a body that is kept on a raw food cleansing diet will initially lose weight rapidly, but eventually weight loss slows to virtually nothing and then stabilizes. However, long-term raw fooders are usually thin as toothpicks.

Once starchy vegetables like potatoes or winter squash, raw or cooked, or any cereals, raw or cooked, are added to a cleansing diet, the detoxification and healing virtually ceases and it becomes very easy to maintain or even gain weight, particularly if larger quantities of more concentrated foods like seeds and nuts are eaten. Though this diet has ceased to be cleansing, few if any toxins from misdigestion will be produced and health is easy to maintain.

"Raw fooders" are usually people who have healed themselves of a serious disease and ever after continue to maintain themselves on unfired food, almost as a matter of religious belief. They have become convinced that eating only raw, unfired food is the key to extraordinarily long life and supreme good health. When raw fooders wish to perform hard physical work or strenuous exercise, they"ll consume raw nuts and some raw grains such as finely-ground oats soaked overnight in warm water or deliciously sweet "Essene bread," made from slightly sprouted wheat that is then ground wet, made into cakes, and sun baked at temperatures below about 115 degrees Fahrenheit. Essene bread can be purchased in some health food stores. However, little or no healing or detoxification can happen once concentrated energy sources are added to the diet, even raw ones.

CHAPTER 5- LEARN TO EAT ONLY WHEN YOU ARE HUNGRY

If we do this we eat only to supply the demands of the body. We cannot repeat too often the admonition, do not eat if not hungry.

If this plan were followed the present three meals-a-day plan would end. Also the practice of many of eating between meals and in the evening before retiring would cease. For most people real hunger would call for about one meal a day, with occasionally some small amounts of fruit during the day.

Hunger is the "voice of nature" saying to us that food is required. There is no other true guide as to when to eat. The time of day, the habitual meal time, etc., are not true guides.

Although genuine hunger is a mouth and throat sensation and depends upon an actual physiological need for food, muscular contractions of the stomach accompany hunger and are thought by physiologists, to give rise to the hunger sensation.

Carlson, of the Chicago University, found that in a man who had been fasting two weeks, these gastric "hunger" contractions had not decreased, although there was no desire for food. The same has been observed in animals. Indeed these contractions are seen to increase and yet they do not produce the sensation of hunger. I do not consider these so-called "hunger-contractions" as the cause of hunger. Real hunger is a mouth and throat sensation.

But there is a difference between hunger and what is called appetite. Appetite is a counterfeit hunger, a creature of habit and cultivation, and may be due to any one of a number of things; such as the arrival of the habitual meal time, the sight, taste, or smell of food, condiments and seasonings, or even the thought of food. In some diseased states there is an almost constant and insatiable appetite. None of these things can arouse true hunger; for, this comes only when there is an actual need for food.

One may have an appetite for tobacco, coffee, tea, opium, alcohol, etc., but he can never be hungry for these, since they serve no real physiological need.

Appetite is often accompanied by a gnawing or "all gone" sensation in the stomach, or a general sense of weakness; there may even be mental depression. Such symptoms usually belong to the diseased stomach of a glutton and will pass away if their owner will refrain from eating for a few days. They are temporarily relieved by eating and this leads to the idea that it was food that was needed. But such sensations and feelings do not accompany true hunger. In true hunger one is not aware that he has a stomach for this, like thirst, is a mouth and throat sensation. Real hunger arises spontaneously, that is without the agency of some external factor, and is accompanied by a "watering of the mouth" and usually by a conscious desire for some particular food.

Dr. Gibson says that, "The condition known as appetite, ... with its source and center in nervous desire, and its motive in self-indulgence, is a mere parasite on life, feeding on its host--the man himself--whose misdirected imagination invites it into his own vital household; while hunger, on the other hand, is the original, constitutional prompter for the cell-world calling for means to supply the true need and necessities of man's physical nature.

Appetite does not express our needs, but our wants; not what we really need, but what we think we need. It is imagination running riot, fashioning out of our gluttonous greed an insatiable vampire which grows with our wants, and increases its power until finally it kills us unless we determine to kill it. ... As long as our attention is absorbed in the pleasures of the table, in the gratification of eating for its own sake, and in the introduction of new combinations to bring about stimulating effects, we are increasing the power of our appetite at the expense of our hunger."

The hungry person is able to eat and relish a crust of dry bread; he who has only an appetite must have his food seasoned and spiced before he can enjoy it. Even a gourmand is able to enjoy a hearty meal if there is sufficient seasoning to whip up his jaded appetite and arouse his palsied taste. He would be far better off if he would await the arrival of hunger before eating.

There is no doubt of the truth of Dr. Geo. S. Weger's thought that "appetite contractions in the stomach are often excited by psychic states, as influenced by the senses." Appetite contractions thus aroused, are of distinct advantage in digesting a meal if they are super-added to pre- existing hunger contractions. We know that these psychic states increase the flow of the digestive juices--make the stomach "water" as well as the mouth--and enhance digestion.

Dr. Claunch says, "the difference between true hunger and false craving may be determined as follows: when hungry and comfortable it is true hunger. When hungry and uncomfortable it is false craving. When a sick person misses a customary meal, he gets weak before he gets hungry. When a healthy person misses a customary meal, he gets hungry before he gets weak."

If we follow the rule to eat only when truly hungry, those people who are "hungry" but weak and uncomfortable would fast until comfort and strength returned. Fasting would become one of the most common practices in our lives, at least, until we learn to live and eat to keep well and thus eliminate the need for fasting.

There are individuals who are always eating and always "hungry." They mistake a morbid irritation of the stomach for hunger. These people have not learned to distinguish between a normal demand for food and a symptom of disease. They mistake the evidences of chronic gastritis or of gastric neurosis for hunger.

Hunger, as previously pointed out, is the insistent demand for food that arises out of physiological need for nourishment. Appetite, on the other hand, is a craving for food which may be the result of several different outside factors operating through the mind and senses. Anything that will arouse an appetite will encourage one to eat, whether or not there is an actual need for food.

Hunger may be satisfied and appetite still persist, a not unusual thing. Our many course dinners, with everything especially prepared to appeal to the taste and smell, are well designed to keep alive appetite, long after hunger has been appeased. No man is ever hungry when he reaches the dessert, so commonly served after a many course dinner. Few, though filled to repletion and perhaps uncomfortable in the abdomen, ever refuse to eat the dessert. It is especially prepared to appeal to appetite. This style of eating necessarily and inevitably leads to overeating and disease. Too many articles of food at a meal over stimulate and induce overeating.

Hunger and the sense of taste are the only guides as to the quantity and character of food required. If we eat when we are not hungry, and if the delicate sensibilities of taste have been dulled and deadened by gluttonous indulgence and by condiments, spices, alcohol, etc., it ceases to be a reliable guide.

The unperverted instinct of hunger craves most keenly the food that is most needed by the body and the unperverted taste derives the most pleasure and satisfaction out of the food or foods demanded, and will be satisfied when we have consumed sufficient of such food or foods to supply the body's needs. But, if we have been in the habit of crowding the stomach when there is no demand for food, just because it is meal time, or because the doctor ordered it, and we know no other indication that enough food has been consumed, than that the stomach can hold no more, we are headed for disaster. The existence of a natural demand for food indicates that food is required by the body and that the organs of the body are ready to receive and digest it. Eating when there is no time, or as a social duty, or because one has been able to stimulate an appetite, is a wrong to the body. Both the quality and quantity, and the frequency of meals should be regulated by the rules of hygiene rather than by those of etiquette and convenience.

CHAPTER 6- FANTASTIC SMOOTHIE RECIPES FOR ATHLETES

Amazing Apple Smoothie

2 cups apple sauce 1 cup apple cider

1 cup orange juice

2 tablespoons Vermont maple syrup 1/2 teaspoons nutmeg

1/2 teaspoons cinnamon

Combine all ingredients in a blender and blend until smooth. Pour into glasses and serve.

Apple Carrot Quencher

Smoothies for Athletes and Weight Loss
2 cups carrot juice 1/2 cups apple juice

6 ounces non-fat vanilla or plain yogurt, frozen 1 banana

Put all ingredients into blender. Blend until smoothie consistency is reached!

Apples and Cream Smoothie

2 cups vanilla low-fat ice cream 1 cup unsweetened applesauce

1/4 teaspoons ground cinnamon or apple pie spice 1 cup fat free skim or 1% low fat milk

Ground cinnamon (optional)

In a blender container combine low-fat ice cream, applesauce, and the 1/4 teaspoons cinnamon or apple pie spice. Cover and blend until smooth. Add fat free skim or 1% low fat milk. Cover and blend until just mixed. Pour into glasses. If desired, sprinkle each serving with additional cinnamon. Serve immediately.

Makes 4 (8-ounces) servings.

Apple Pie Smoothie

1 frozen banana

1/2 peeled, chopped apple 1 cup apple juice

1/2 teaspoons cinnamon Pinch of nutmeg

Blend. Great substitute for applesauce! Control the consistency by adding more or less chopped apple.

Jared Boulder
Apricot Apple Smoothie

1 apple (golden delicious), peeled, cored & chopped 1 cup apple juice

4 apricots, fresh, pitted (skin optional) 1 banana, peeled

3/4 cups yogurt, plain 10 - 12 ice cubes

1 tablespoon honey

Place all ingredients in a blender and puree until smooth.

Arctic Forest Smoothie

1 peach, frozen

10 blueberries, frozen

1 cup light (reduced sugar) fat-free vanilla yogurt, frozen 1/2 cups 1% milk

1/2 tablespoons crushed pecan 1/2 teaspoons salt

1/4 teaspoons vanilla extract

Put all ingredients into blender. Blend until smoothie consistency is reached!

Avocado Avalanche

1 large avocado

2 teaspoons condensed milk 1 cup ice

Scoop out avocado into blender. Add 2 teaspoons condensed milk or a little more, depending on how sweet you like it. Then add the ice and blend all of it together until it's a semi-creamy texture.

Avocado Banana Berry Smoothie

Half a ripe avocado

1 to 1 1/2 frozen bananas

4 to 5 frozen or fresh strawberries Splash non-fat soy or other nut milk Pinch cardamom

Pinch allspice

Whatever else strikes your fancy. . . Nuts, fruits, spices, etc throw all ingredients into a blender and blend until desired texture is reached. I prefer it smooth, but some like a chewable drink. Very, very delicious! Serves: 1

Banana Blueberry Smoothie

2 bananas

1/2 cups blueberries 1 cup plain yogurt

Peel bananas, slice and place on a cookie sheet. Put in freezer and freeze until solid. Remove from freezer and place in blender. Slice berries and add to blender. Pour in yogurt. Blend until smooth. Pour into glass and serve.

Banana Hazelnut Smoothie

4 medium bananas, peeled and sliced into 1/2 inch pieces 6 tablespoons light brown sugar

Jared Boulder
1/4 cups hazelnuts 1 cup ice cubes 1/4 cups milk

1/4 cups dark rum or hazelnut liqueur

2 tablespoons chopped hazelnuts, for garnish (optional)

Place the sliced bananas in a sealed plastic bag and put them in the freezer for 1 hour. Place the brown sugar and 1/4 cups hazelnuts in a blender and grind together until fine. Place the frozen bananas, ice cubes, milk, and rum in the blender with the sugar and nut mixture. Blend until smooth. Pour the smoothies into 4 goblets or tall glasses. Garnish with chopped nuts, if desired. Serve immediately.

Banana Nut bread Smoothie

1 ounce hazelnut liqueur ounces banana liqueur ounces vanilla syrup

2 ounces half and half banana

2 cups of ice

1 teaspoon chopped walnuts 2 ounces whipped cream

Pour liqueurs, syrup, half and half, banana and half of the walnuts into blender. Add ice and blend until smooth. Pour into glass and top with whipped cream. Sprinkle chopped nuts on top.

Banana Oatmeal Smoothie

1 cup milk

1 packet instant oatmeal, regular flavor 1 whole banana, cut in chunks

Smoothies for Athletes and Weight Loss
1 cup orange juice

Combine all ingredients in a blender. Cover and blend on high speed for 1 minute.

Banana Orange Twist

3 ounces frozen orange juice concentrate 1/4 teaspoons vanilla

1/2 cups milk 1/2 cups water

1/2 small banana, sliced 5 ice cubes

Combine everything except ice and blend for 15 seconds. Add ice and blend for 2 minutes.

Banana Pearberry Smoothie

1 medium banana

1 cup pear nectar (Goya brand is very good)

1 tablespoon seedless raspberry jam (use Polaner all-fruit if possible) 6 ice cubes or. . . 1 cup of ice

Place all ingredients into a blender. Blend on high speed until all of the ice has dissolved and the consistency is smooth, about 2 minutes.

Banana Split Smoothie

1 cup nonfat milk

1 1/2 cups frozen banana slices 1/2 cups pineapple chunks

5 frozen strawberries

1 1/2 to 2 tablespoons sweetened cocoa powder (to taste)

Pour milk into the blender first. Add cocoa and then fruit. Put cover on and blend until smooth.

Basic Fruit Smoothie

1 quarter strawberries, hulled 1 banana, broken into chunks 2 peaches

1 cup orange or peach or mango or apple juice 2 cups ice

In a blender, combine strawberries, banana and peaches. Blend until fruit is pureed. Blend in the juice. Add ice and blend to desired consistency. Pour into glasses and serve.

Berry Almond Blast

1/2 cups frozen whole berries (use blackberries, strawberries or raspberries) 1 cup nonfat soy milk

3/4 teaspoons almond extract

1/2 cups silken tofu (about 4 ounces) 2 tablespoons granulated sugar

Combine all ingredients in blender and blend until smooth. Makes 2 smoothies.

Berry Banana Smoothie

1 large banana, peeled, sliced and frozen

3/4 cups frozen or fresh strawberries, raspberries or blueberries 3/4 cups low- or non-fat vanilla frozen yogurt

1 12ounces can or bottle of regular or diet ginger ale, chilled

Place all the ingredients in a blender or food processor. Cover and blend at highest speed until smooth. Note: if you use fresh berries, try to use a frozen banana, and if you use a fresh banana, go for frozen berries. Otherwise your drink will be too thin. Both fruits being frozen will give you a satisfyingly thick drink.

Berry Bliss Smoothie

2 scoops raspberry sherbet

4 strawberries

15 blueberries

5 blackberries

16 ounces orange juice (or juice of your choice)

Put all ingredients in a blender, juice last, then blend until smooth. To add thickness try adding more sherbet or ice to the smoothie. Pour Into a tall glass to serve.

Berry Blue Smoothie

2 cups fresh or slightly thawed frozen blueberries 1 (8-ounces) container low fat vanilla yogurt

1 (6-ounces) cups milk

1 (12-ounces) can pineapple juice 3 tablespoons honey

12 to 16 ice cubes

Jared Boulder

Place all ingredients, except the ice cubes, into container of electric blender and blend on high until smooth. With blender running, add 2 to 3 ice cubes at a time through the center opening in the lid until all ice cubes have been added. Blend until smooth. Serve immediately. Makes 4 servings.

Beta Carotene Blast

3 small ice cubes

2 apricots (sliced and pitted) 1/2 papaya (frozen in chunks)

1/2 mango (frozen in chunks) 1/2 cups carrot juice

1 tablespoon honey

Add ingredients (except for honey) to blender in the order listed, and then blend on high speed for 30 seconds. Add honey and blend a few seconds more. Serve in a frosted glass. Option: add orange juice for a thinner consistency.

Black And Blue Bomber

1/4 cups blueberries 1/4 cups blackberries 1 banana

1/2 cups apple juice

1/3 cups raspberry sorbet

Put all ingredients into blender. Blend until smoothie consistency is reached!

Blackberry Smoothie

3/4 cups apple juice 1/2 cups plain yogurt

1 1/2 cups frozen blackberries 1 banana

Pour liquid ingredients into the blender first. Yogurt is a liquid ingredient. All fruit goes into blender at one time. Put cover on and blend until smooth.

Blueberry Smoothie

1/2 bag of frozen blueberries

2 tablespoons blueberry preserves 7 or 8 ice cubes

1 1/2 cups of soymilk 1 banana

This is super easy. Just toss everything into a blender, switch to the highest setting, and let fly until you stop hearing ice cubes crunching and everything is fairly smooth. There are an infinite number of variations on this using different combinations of fruit and jam. You might also consider adding protein powder, ground flax seed, or any other supplement that strikes your fancy. It's best to wait until near the end, and just blend long enough to mix the protein powder of whatever in. You can also substitute apple juice for the soymilk to create a tangier concoction.

Blueberry Banana Smoothie

1 banana, preferably frozen

A handful of blueberries, frozen or fresh

1 cup of milk reduced fat or skim milk (or soy milk) Combine in a blender or with a hand blender. Enjoy!

Blueberry Maple Smoothie

Jared Boulder

1 cup low-fat blueberry yogurt 3/4 cups low-fat milk

1 tablespoon maple syrup 1/2 teaspoons cinnamon

2 cups fresh blueberries, frozen

Combine the yogurt, milk, syrup, and cinnamon in a blender. Add the blueberries and blend until smooth.

Blueberry Orange Smoothie

12 ounces frozen blueberries, unthawed. . . Or. . . 2 1/2 cups fresh blueberries 8 ounces vanilla low fat yogurt

1/2 cups orange juice 1/2 cups milk

1 teaspoon vanilla extract

Whirl all ingredients together in a blender until smooth. Serve immediately.

Cappuccino Smoothie

2 cups brewed double strength coffee 1 pint coffee ice cream

6 cups ice

1 1/2 cups milk   Whipped cream, if desired Cinnamon for garnish

Place coffee, ice cream, ice and milk in blender. Mix until smooth. Top with whipped cream and cinnamon.

Carob Smoothie

3-4 dates, pitted and soaked 20 minutes 1 cup nut or grain milk

Smoothies for Athletes and Weight Loss
1 frozen banana, cut in chunks 3-4 tablespoons carob powder Dash vanilla (optional)

Place dates in a small bowl with just enough water to cover. Let them soak 20 minutes, drain. In blender, combine the dates, nut milk, banana, carob powder and vanilla. Blend until smooth. Drink immediately.

Cherry Berry Smoothie

1 cup low-fat cherry yogurt

1/4 cups cranberry juice

1 cup frozen, pitted cherries

3/4 cups frozen, unsweetened blueberries

Combine the yogurt and cranberry juice in a blender. Add the cherries and berries. Blend until smooth. Makes about 2-1/2 cups, serves 2.

Cherry Cantaloupe Smoothie

1/2 cantaloupe (peeled, seeded, and sliced) 1/2 cups apple or apricot juice

2-3 pitted cherries

1/4 cups raspberries or blackberries 3-4 ice cubes

Put all ingredients into blender. Blend until smoothie consistency is reached!

Cherry Vanilla Smoothie

Jared Boulder
1 cup frozen vanilla yogurt

1 cup apple juice

2 cups frozen cherries

Pour liquid ingredients into the blender first. Yogurt is a liquid ingredient. Add cherries. Put cover on and blend until smooth.

Chocolate Banana Smoothie

1 frozen banana -- peeled

6 ounces light (reduced sugar) fat-free vanilla or cherry frozen yogurt 2 tablespoons Hershey s chocolate syrup

1/2 cups non-fat milk

Put all ingredients into blender. Blend until smoothie consistency is reached!

Chocolate Mint Smoothie

4 scoops peppermint ice cream 1 1/2 cups milk

2 drops peppermint extract 1 teaspoon vanilla extract

4 tablespoons bittersweet chocolate syrup

Combine in a blender container and blend until no white shows. Serve immediately.

Chocolate Peanut Butter Banana Smoothie

1/2 cups rice milk 1/2 cups silken tofu

Smoothies for Athletes and Weight Loss
1/3 cups creamy peanut butter

2 fresh bananas, frozen and sliced

2 tablespoons chocolate syrup 6 ice cubes

Combine the rice milk, tofu and peanut butter in a blender. Add the bananas, chocolate syrup and ice cubes. Blend until smooth, about 30 to 40 seconds. Makes 2 servings.

Citrus Cooler

6 1/2 cups ruby red or pink grapefruit juice, divided 2 cups pineapple juice

1 (6 ounces) can frozen orange juice concentrate, thawed and undiluted 2 cups lime-flavored sparkling mineral water, chilled

Garnish: lime slices

Pour 2 1/2 cups grapefruit juice into ice trays, filling 28 sections, freeze. Combine remaining 4 cups grapefruit juice, pineapple juice, and orange juice concentrate, stir well. Cover and chill at least 3 hours. Stir in mineral water just before serving. Place 3 frozen grapefruit juice cubes in each of 9 glasses, fill each fruit juice mixture. Garnish, if desired. Serve immediately.

Citrus Tea Smoothie

1 cup orange segments, chilled

1/2 cups grapefruit segments, chilled

1/2 cups strong-brewed earl grey tea, chilled 3/4 cups orange sherbet

Jared Boulder
2 ice cubes, crushed

Combine the orange segments, grapefruit segments, and tea in a blender. Add the sherbet and ice. Blend until smooth.

Cocoa Berry Smoothie

3/4 cups apple juice 1 cup vanilla yogurt

2 cups mixed frozen berries

2 to 3 tablespoons sweetened powdered cocoa

Pour liquid ingredients into the blender first. Yogurt is a liquid ingredient. Add berries and cocoa. Put cover on and blend until smooth.

Coconut Ginger Smoothie

1/4 cups apple juice

1 pinch coconut, grated or. . . 1 tablespoon coconut milk * 1/2 banana

1/4 teaspoons ginger root -- fresh, peeled, grated 1/2 cups crushed ice -- or 2 small ice cubes

* can be made from fresh or dried coconut or purchased bottled. Do not use the canned coconut mix for mixed drinks as it is very sweet and different. If using fresh coconut, cut coconut meat into 1" pieces & place equal amounts of coconut & hot water in food processor or blender. Puree at high speed for a couple of minutes, let steep for 30 minutes.

Pour into a strainer set over a bowl. Press on the pulp and squeeze by the handful to extract as milk as possible. Pour the milk through a fine-mesh strainer. For dried coconut: use 1 cup p unsweetened, dried coconut with 1 1/2 cups hot tap water. Allow to stand for 5 minutes. Puree one minute and proceed as above. Will keep up to three days refrigerated and indefinitely, if frozen. Blend all ingredients in a blender or food processor until smooth.

Coffee Smoothie

3 to 4 tablespoons instant coffee powder 1 cup milk (nonfat okay)

1 cup vanilla frozen yogurt

1 cup frozen bananas

Pour liquid ingredients into the blender first. Yogurt is a liquid ingredient. Add bananas. Put cover on and blend until smooth.

Cucumber Mint Smoothie

1 cucumber, peeled, seeded and chopped

3 tablespoons mint leaves & mint sprigs -- finely chopped 1 1/2 cups apple juice or still cider

1 cup lemon sorbet

1 cup ice cubes

Place the cucumber, mint, apple juice or cider, sorbet and ice in a blender, and blend until smooth. Garnish with mint, and serve.

Daiquiri Twist Smoothie

Jared Boulder
1 cup apple-cranberry juice 1/2 cups orange juice

1/2 cups frozen blackberries 1/2 cups kiwis

1/2 cups crushed ice 1/2 teaspoons sugar

1 scoop vanilla ice cream

Place ingredients in a blender and puree until smooth.

Date Yogurt Smoothie

1/2 cups chopped dates

1 banana, chopped, (about 1/2 cup) 1/2 cups orange juice

1/2 cups plain nonfat yogurt 1/2 cups crushed ice

Combine dates, banana slices, and orange juice in a blender and puree until dates are finely chopped. Add yogurt and ice, blend until just combined.

Double Apple Smoothie

2 bananas

1 green apple

1 red apple

10-12 frozen strawberries 1-2 cups apple juice

Put all the ingredients in the blender in the order listed and mix on high until fully blended.

Double Melon Smoothie

Smoothies for Athletes and Weight Loss
1 1/2 cups seeded and chopped watermelon

1 1/2 cups seeded and chopped honeydew melon Juice of 2 limes

1 cup vanilla low fat yogurt

1 cup ice cubes

Place all ingredients in a blender and blend until smooth. Pour into glasses.

CHAPTER 7- BONUS SMOOTHIE RECIPES

Everything but the Kitchen Sink Smoothie

2 bananas 1 orange 1 apple

2 chunks of fresh pineapple 2 kiwis

1/2 cups of frozen blueberries 10-12 frozen strawberries 1-2 cups cranberry juice

1 (14-ounces) can eagle brand sweetened condensed milk (not evaporated milk) 1 (8-ounces) carton plain yogurt

1 small banana, cut up

1 cup frozen or fresh whole strawberries

1 (8-ounces) can crushed pineapple packed with juice, chilled 2 tablespoons real lemon juice from concentrate

1 cup ice cubes

Halved fresh strawberries, optional

Chill eagle brand. In blender container, combine eagle brand, yogurt, banana, whole strawberries, pineapple with its juice and real lemon, cover and blend until smooth. With blender running, gradually add ice cubes, blending until smooth. Garnish with halved strawberries if desired. Serve immediately.

Flaxseed Smoothie

1 medium banana or fruit of choice 1/4 cups yogurt or tofu

1 to 2 tablespoons concentrated fruit juice 1/4 teaspoons vanilla

1/3 cups soy milk

1 tablespoon flaxseed oil   1 tablespoon flaxseed meal Dash cinnamon or mace

Blend all together until creamy smooth.

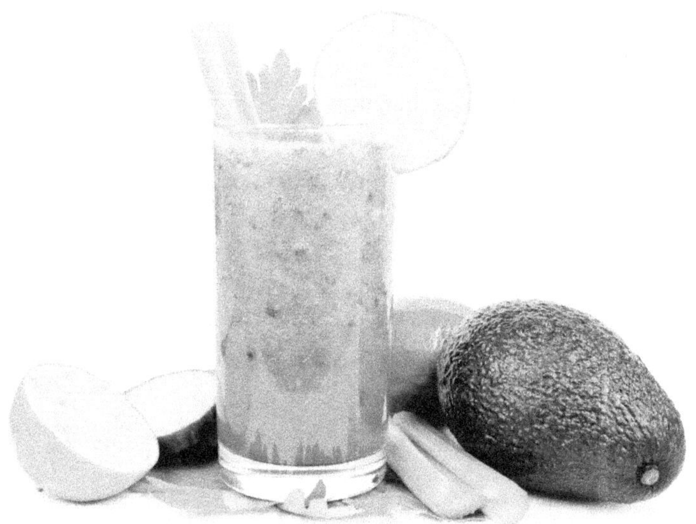

Frosty Fruit Smoothie With Wheat Germ

1 cup low-fat vanilla yogurt

1 cup sliced peaches, fresh, frozen or canned 1 ripe banana, cut into chunks

1/4 cups wheat germ 1/4 cups orange juice 1 cup ice cubes

Peach or banana slices, opt. 2 teaspoons wheat germ, optional

In blender or food processor, combine yogurt, peaches, banana, wheat germ, 1/4 cups orange juice and ice cubes. Cover and blend about 1 minute, or until smooth. Serve immediately, poured into tall glasses and garnished with peach or banana slices and sprinkled with 2 teaspoons wheat germ.

Frozen Fruit Smoothie

1/2 cups frozen bananas   1/2 cups frozen peaches   1/2 cups frozen strawberries 2 cups milk

1/4 cups orange juice 2 tablespoons honey

In a blender, combine all the above until smooth. Pour in tall glasses, pop a straw in and enjoy! Wonderful for those hot days in the summertime.

Fruit Cocktail Smoothie

8 ounces canned fruit cocktail, chilled

1 cup milk

1/4 cups nonfat dry milk powder 1/2 teaspoons vanilla

1/2 cups ice cubes

2 dashes ground cinnamon

In a blender container combine undrained fruit cocktail and remaining ingredients. Cover, blend till combined. Add ice cubes, cover and blend till smooth. Sprinkle with additional cinnamon (for garnish) if desired. Serve immediately.

Fruit Salad Smoothie

1 medium ripe peach

3/4 cups fresh or frozen strawberries 1/2 banana -- peeled

2 cups skimmed evaporated milk -chilled   4 teaspoons frozen orange juice concentrate 1 teaspoon vanilla

4-6 ice cubes Cinnamon -- optional

Combine everything in blender except ice and cinnamon. With blender running, add ice cubes one at a time. Divide smoothie into 4 chilled glasses and sprinkle with cinnamon.

Fruity Sunflower Smoothie

1/3 20ounces bag frozen strawberries 1 banana

1/2 15ounces can pineapple (including juice), or several slices of fresh pineapple 3 tablespoons low-fat plain yogurt

2 tablespoons unsalted sunflower seeds 6 ounces orange juice

Blend for about 30 seconds, and then serve.

Gingerroot Smoothie

1 apple, cored, peeled, and sliced 1 lemon, peeled and seeded

1/2 cups filtered water 1/2 cups ice

1 (2-inch) piece fresh gingerroot, peeled and crushed

This is a good smoothie for a queasy tummy. Drink it slowly. Blend all ingredients until smooth.

Granola Peach Smoothie

Jared Boulder

1 ripe, medium-size peach 2 teaspoons lemon juice 2 teaspoons honey

1/2 cups yogurt

2 tablespoons granola or buckwheat crunchies

Blend the first four ingredients. Sprinkle granola or buckwheat on top.

Grape Cherry Guzzler

2 cups 100% grape juice from concord grapes (bottled or frozen reconstituted) 2 tablespoons lemon juice

1 cup frozen dark sweet pitted cherries 1/2 teaspoons cinnamon

1/2 cups plain nonfat yogurt

Process all in blender until smooth. Pour over crushed ice.

Grapefruit Smoothie

1 large grapefruit, peeled and sectioned

1 8ounces container vanilla, orange or apricot-flavored low fat yogurt 2 teaspoons sugar

4 ice cubes

Fresh mint for garnish (optional)

In blender container, place grapefruit sections, yogurt, and sugar. Cover and blend on medium speed. While machine is running, add ice cubes one at a time through hole in cover, cover and blend for

45 to 60 seconds at high speed until frothy. If desired, to remove pulp, pour through strainer to serve. Garnish with fresh mint if desired.

Guava Smoothie

1 frozen banana

1 cup of frozen strawberries

1 cup peach sorbet

1 can guava nectar Blend until smooth.

Hawaiian Silk Smoothie

1 cup soy milk

1/2 cups pineapple juice 1 frozen banana

1 tablespoon maple syrup

2 tablespoons nonfat dry milk Ice cubes

1 tablespoon coconut milk

Put all ingredients into blender. Blend until smoothie consistency is reached!

Holiday Punch Smoothie

2 cups orange juice 2 cups lemon juice

2 cups grenadine syrup 3 quarts ginger ale

1 pint of quartered strawberries or sliced fruit in season

Mix juices and syrup. Pour over block of ice to chill. Just before serving, add ginger ale and fruit.

Tofu Fruit Smoothie

1/2 cups apple juice

1/2 cups frozen vanilla nonfat yogurt, or any flavor of sorbet 4 ounces (1/2 cup) soft tofu, drained

1 cup fresh or frozen sliced strawberries or peaches 1 banana, peeled and broken into chunks

1 teaspoon honey 1/2 cups ice cubes

Fresh whole berries for garnish (optional)

Place all ingredients into container of electric blender. Blend on high until smooth, about 30 seconds.

Tropical Fling Smoothie

1/2 cups each ripe pineapple and mango, cut up 1/2 cups milk

1/2 cups plain yogurt

2 teaspoons fresh lime juice

Process ingredients in blender or food processor until smooth and sweeten to taste.

Tropical Fruit Smoothie

1 cup frozen honeydew melon

1 cup frozen mango

Smoothies for Athletes and Weight Loss
1 frozen banana

1 cup plain yogurt

8 ounces peach nectar

Blend until smooth. Serves two.

Tropical Strawberry Smoothie

1 cup guava nectar

1 cup pineapple chunks   3/4 cups frozen peaches   3/4 cups frozen strawberries

Pour guava nectar into the blender first. All fruit goes into blender at one time. Put cover on and blend until smooth.

Ultimate Smoothie

1 cup fresh-squeezed orange juice Flesh of 2 mangos

8 ounces (small package) of fresh or frozen blueberries 1 frozen banana

2 tablespoons flax seeds

1 teaspoon honey or maple syrup

Put all the ingredients in the blender in the order listed and mix on high until fully blended.

Vitamin Cups Smoothie

2 bananas 1 orange 2 kiwis

Jared Boulder
10-12 frozen strawberries   1/2 cups of frozen blueberries 1-2 cups of orange juice

Put all the ingredients in the blender in the order listed and mix on high until fully blended.

Wacky Watermelon Smoothie

2 cups seeded watermelon chunks 1 cup cracked ice

1/2 cups plain yogurt 1 tablespoon sugar

1/2 teaspoons ground ginger 1/8 teaspoons almond extract

Combine all ingredients in blender container, blend until smooth.

Zippy Pineapple Carrot Smoothie

1/2 cups pineapple chunks 1 cup soy milk, any flavor 1 carrot, peeled and sliced 1/3 cups pineapple juice

1-1" piece ginger (peeled and minced) Honey to taste

Place all ingredients in blender container and blend until everything is smooth. Add ice if you like it frosty. The ginger adds the "zip".

ABOUT THE AUTHOR

Jared Boulder is not an athlete by any means but he has always had an interest in eating healthy. Athletes are always on a healthy diet and have to maintain a strict regimen to be able to perform at their best. He was not the best at dieting and found that having a nutrient packed smoothie or fruit juice would keep him going until it was time to have the next meal.

That is how he started having the same types of smoothies with were recommended for athletes. They were not only healthier options but filled with the necessary nutrients. That is what he is advising others of in his book.